The Pa Protocol

A Quick Reference Guide of Foods
To Include and Eliminate in
The Paleo AIP

by
Anne Angelone

Disclaimer

This manual is not intended to provide medical
advice or to take the place of medical advice and
treatment from your personal physician. Readers
are advised to consult their own doctors or other
qualified health professionals regarding the
treatment of medical conditions. The author, shall
not be held liable or responsible for any
misunderstanding or misuse of the information
contained in this program manual or for any loss,
damage, or injury caused or alleged to be caused
directly or indirectly by any treatment, action, or
application of any food or food source discussed in
this program manual. The U.S. Food and Drug
Administration have not evaluated the statements
in this program manual. This information is not
intended to diagnose, treat, cure, or prevent any
disease. To request permission for reproduction or
inquire about private classes, please contact:

Anne Angelone, MS, Licensed Acupuncturist
www.anneangelone.com

Table of Contents

The Premise:

Eliminating known inflammatory foods, resolving dysbiosis, SIBO et al. infections while healing the mucosal lining and strengthening gut immunity, are the keys to optimal health and balanced immune function. The terms "autoimmune paleo", "the autoimmune protocol" or "AIP" have come to refer to a food plan geared toward improving immune function via decreasing triggers, strengthening digestion, and improving overall health. The goal is to increase anti-inflammatory superfoods to heal the integrity of the gut lining while simultaneously eliminating foods that create low grade immune/inflammatory responses, irritate the gut lining, and feed harmful bacteria (which lead to SIBO and dysbiosis). By eliminating the underlying mechanisms that drive inflammation and autoimmunity, you can modulate and bring balance to your overactive immune system.

The current protocol includes superfoods to eat on a daily basis along with probiotic and cultured foods to promote healthy intestinal micro-flora and strengthen gut immunity. The AIP serves as an excellent template to rapidly reduce inflammation and heal intestinal permeability also via specific dietary interventions. The list of foods to avoid also notes potential suspect foods including FODMAPS, high oxalate, histamine and salicylate foods and foods that contribute to SIBO.

To calm down the immune/inflammatory response and allow the gut to heal, it is suggested to remove the major offending foods: eggs, grains, alcohol, nightshades, nuts, seeds, legumes, and dairy et al. items on the "Foods To Eliminate" list for at least 30 days. It is recommended to use this dietary template for 30 days and continue on it for longer especially if re-introduced foods cause any reactions. It is suggested to inform your health care provider of your dietary changes and of any exacerbation of symptoms if reintroducing foods.

The AIP emphasis on whole, organic, and nutrient dense foods contributes to optimal digestion and immune function with anti-inflammatory and antioxidant rich fruit and vegetables. Blood sugar will stabilize and adrenals will strengthen with lots of minerals and amino acids from both protein and veggies.

The Paleo Autoimmune Protocol sets the foundation for halting autoimmune reactions. This book is meant as a handy reference guide of foods to include and avoid while on the protocol. For fabulous recipes, there is a thriving online community of excellent people dedicated to making this a very delicious experience. For satisfying recipes, please find links to these resources at the end of this e-book.

Many thanks and tons of gratitude to Sarah Ballantyne, Ph.D., aka The Paleo Mom for editing and contributing to the food lists in this manual and for inspiring a very healthy direction to all. For more information on the science behind the AIP, please read Sarah's book: The Paleo Approach: Reverse Autoimmune Disease and Heal Your Body, due out in the very near future.

	FOODS TO INCLUDE In The Autoimmune Protocol	FOODS TO ELIMINATE In The Autoimmune Protocol
FRUITS	Apples, apricots, Asian pears, bananas, blueberries, blackberry, boysenberry, cherries, cranberry, figs, grapefruit, kiwi, lemons, limes, melons, nectarine, oranges, peaches, pears, persimmons, plums, pluots, plantains, pomegranate, raspberry, strawberry.

Caution: high glycemic fruits: watermelon, mango, pineapple, raisins, grapes, dried fruit, dehydrated fruit.

FODMAPs: Apples, apricots, cherries, nectarines, peaches, pears, persimmon, plum, pluots. | **Avoid**: canned fruits.

SIBO caution: Plantains, green bananas.

FODMAPs: Apples, apricots, cherries, nectarines, peaches, pears, persimmon, plum, pluots. |

limit

Suspect foods →

5

| VEGETABLES 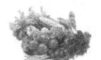 | Asparagus, artichoke hearts, arugula, avocado, basil, beet, beet greens, broccoli, broccoli rabe, Brussels sprouts, burdock, bok choy, cabbage, carrots, cauliflower, celery, chard, chicory, collards, chard, cucumber, daikon, dandelion greens, fennel root, green cabbage, Jerusalem artichoke, jicama, kale, kohlrabi, leeks, lettuce, mustard, Napa cabbage, nettles, okra, onions, parsnips, pumpkin, purslane, radish, radicchio, red cabbage scallion, spinach, shallot, summer squash, turnips, water chestnuts, watercress, zucchini.

FODMAPs:
Artichoke, asparagus, avocado, beet root, broccoli, Brussels sprouts, butternut squash, all cabbage, cauliflower, celery, fennel | Avoid:
Nightshades:
Potatoes (not sweet potatoes), all tomatoes, green peppers, chili peppers, eggplants, tomatillos, sweet bell peppers, jalapenos, cayenne, habanero, Anaheim and Serrano, chili peppers in dried powders such as paprika, chili powder, curry powder, cayenne, hot sauces, salsas, goji berries, ashwaganda, tobacco.

SIBO caution:
parsnips, jicama, kohlrabi, okra, sweet potato, yams, Jerusalem artichoke, parsnips.

FODMAPs:
Artichoke, asparagus, avocado, beet root, broccoli, Brussels sprouts, butternut squash, all cabbage, cauliflower, celery, fennel bulb, garlic, leeks, mushrooms, okra, onions, pumpkin, radicchio, sauerkraut. |

	bulb, garlic, leeks, mushrooms, okra, onions, pumpkin, radicchio, sauerkraut.	
DENSE CARBS 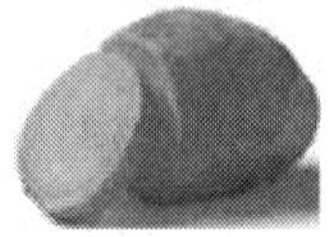	Acorn squash, beets, butternut squash, plantain, lotus root, sweet potato, taro, yams. cassava root, manioc, tapioca, yucca. *FODMAPs:* Butternut squash, sweet potatoes,yams.	*SIBO caution:* Sweet potato, yams, taro, cassava root, manioc, tapioca, yucca, plantain, lotus root. *FODMAPs:* Butternut squash, sweet potatoes, yams.
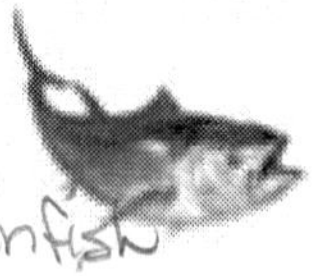 **WILD FISH**	Salmon, mackerel, herring, halibut, shellfish, oysters, cod, tuna, flounder, sardines, hake, skate, trout, red snapper, etc.	**Avoid:** Whale, shark, swordfish. Farmed tilapia and catfish quantities should be moderate.
MEAT 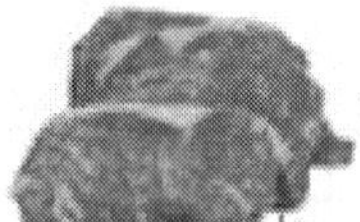	Beef, chicken; quail, squab, duck, goose, turkey, Cornish game hen; pasture-raised lamb, pork, buffalo/bison, goat, emu, ostrich, sausage (without fillers or nightshade spices); liver, kidney, heart, organic sliced meats (gluten, sugar free),	**Avoid:** Processed and canned meats: bacon, fatty cuts of lamb, beef, pork, deli meats, smoked/dried/salted meat and fish. Sausages and deli meats with seed-based or nightshade spices.

(handwritten annotations)

Next to WILD FISH (left margin):
blue fish
Grouper
haddock
mackerel
Perch
Walleye

sunfish

bass, Pike
elk

Next to MEAT:
see back pg for protein + fat %'s
rabbit

eggs

game meat

Bottom of page:
seafood!
abalone
clams
crab

crayfish
lobster
mussels

oysters
scallops
shrimp

	uncured nitrate/nitrite-free deli meats and bacon from grass-fed/pastured beef/pork.	
MILK AND YOGURT	Coconut milk, unsweetened coconut yogurt, unsweetened coconut kefir.	**Avoid:** Coconut yogurt or coconut kefir with sweeteners and/or corn or rice-based thickening agents. *FODMAPs*: dried coconut, coconut flour, coconut cream, coconut milk, and coconut butter.
FATS	Extra virgin olive oil, avocado oil, coconut oil, red palm oil, tallow from grass-fed beef or lamb, lard from pastured pork. *Caution*: nut and seed based oils: flaxseed oil, sesame oil, walnut oil, hazelnut oil, and Macadamia nut oil.	**Avoid:** Margarine, butter, shortening, any processed hydrogenated oils, peanut oil, mayonnaise.
NUTS AND SEEDS		**Avoid:** all nuts and seeds including almonds, Brazil nuts, cashews, chestnuts, hazelnuts, macadamias,

		pecans, walnuts, pine nuts, pistachios, pumpkin seeds, sunflower seeds and seed based spices: anise, annatto, black cumin, celery, coriander, cumin, dill, fennel, fenugreek, mustard, nutmeg, poppy, sesame.
COCONUT	Coconut oil, coconut butter, coconut flour, coconut milk, coconut cream, unsweetened coconut yogurt, coconut kefir, unsweetened coconut flakes, coconut aminos. *FODMAPs*: dried coconut, coconut flour, coconut cream, coconut milk, and coconut butter.	*FODMAPs*: dried coconut, coconut flour, coconut cream, coconut butter and coconut milk.
BEVERAGES	Filtered or distilled water, herbal tea, mineral water, broths, freshly made veggie juice, green smoothies, kefir water, coconut kefir, kombucha.	**Avoid**: Sodas, alcoholic beverages, coffee, tea, or any other caffeinated beverages, fruit juice.

FERMENTED FOODS	Sauerkraut, pickled ginger, pickled cucumbers, coconut yogurt, coconut kefir, kefir water, kombucha, kimchi, pickles fermented with salt, beet kvass, lacto-fermented vegetables and fruits such as fermented beets, carrots, and green papaya.	
HERBS AND SPICES	Ginger, rosemary, basil, cilantro, dill, ginger, lemongrass, peppermint, oregano, parsley, sage, sea, salt, thyme, tarragon, turmeric, spearmint, marjoram, mace, chives, chamomile, chervil, cinnamon, bay leaves, cloves, dill, horseradish, saffron, sea salt.	**Avoid Nightshades:** chili peppers, jalapenos, cayenne, habanero, Anaheim and Serrano, chili peppers in dried powders such as paprika, chili powder, curry powder, cayenne, hot sauces, salsas. *Caution:* black pepper, allspice, white, green and pink peppercorns, juniper, cardamom, star anise, vanilla bean, Garam Masala, Chinese 5 Spice.

SUGAR SUBSTITUTES	Cinnamon, mint and ginger. *Caution:* honey, maple syrup, molasses, unrefined cane sugar, and date sugar.	**Avoid:** white or brown sugar, high fructose corn syrup, corn syrup, fruit sweeteners, Truvia, agave, brown rice syrup, Splenda, Equal, Nutrasweet, Xylitol, stevia, raw green stevia, coconut sugar and palm sugar.
BEANS AND LEGUMES		**Avoid:** all beans, black-eyed peas, cashews, chickpeas, lentils, miso, peas, peanuts/peanut butter, soybean and soy products.
FUNGI	Button mushrooms, oyster, portabella, chanterelle, puffball, crimini, etc. *FODMAPs:* mushrooms	**Avoid:** medicinal mushroom extracts e.g. Shiitake, Reishi and Maitake. *FODMAPs:* mushrooms
SOY		**Avoid:** soy milk, soy sauce, tofu, tempeh, soy protein, and edamame.

CONDIMENTS	Apple cider vinegar, Balsamic vinegar, coconut vinegar, Red Boat fish sauce and coconut aminos.	Avoid: Ketchup, relish, soy sauce, BBQ sauce, chutneys, baker's yeast, brewer's yeast.
GRAINS		Avoid: Amaranth, barley, buckwheat, corn including cornmeal and popcorn, millet, oats, oatmeal, quinoa, rice, rye, sorghum, teff, triticale, and wheat including varieties such as spelt, emmer, farro, einkorn, kamut, durum and forms such as bulgur, cracked wheat and wheat berries.
GRAINS PRODUCTS		Avoid: Corn tortillas, chips, starch, syrup, noodles, cakes, breads, rolls, muffins, noodles, crackers, cookies, cake, doughnuts, pancakes, waffles, pasta, tortillas, pizza, pita/flat bread, all processed foods.

GRAIN LIKE SUBSTANCES OR PSEUDO-CEREALS		**Avoid:** Amaranth, buckwheat, cattail, chia, cockscomb, kañiwa, pitseed, goosefoot, quinoa, and wattleseed aka acacia seed.
GLUTEN CONTAINING FOODS		**Avoid:** BBQ sauce, binders, bouillon, brewer's yeast, cold cuts, condiments, emulsifiers, fillers, gum, hot dogs, hydrolyzed plant and vegetable protein, ketchup, soy sauce, lunch meats, malt, malt flavoring, malt vinegar, matzo, modified food starch, monosodium glutamate, non-dairy creamer, processed salad dressings, seitan, stabilizers, teriyaki sauce, textured vegetable protein.
NIGHTSHADE VEGETABLES		**Avoid:** Eggplant, ashwaganda, goji berries, all potatoes (except sweet potatoes), all tomatoes and peppers e.g. chili peppers, tomatillos, sweet bell peppers, jalapenos, cayenne, Habanero, Anaheim, Serrano, paprika, chili powder, curry powder, cayenne, hot sauces, salsas

		potatoes, endive, asparagus, Brussels sprouts, cucumbers, celery, beets, beet greens, chard.
IMMUNE STIMULATING HERBS, SUPPLEMENTS AND EXTRACTS		*Avoid immune stimulants:* Astragalus, ashwaganda, beta glucans, caffeine, chlorella, coffee, echinacea purpurea extract, genistein, glycyrrhiza, goldenseal, grape seed extract green tea, licorice root, lycopene, Maitake, Melissa officinalis (lemon balm), panax ginseng, pine bark extract, pycnogenol, quercetin, Reishi, Shiitake, willow bark.

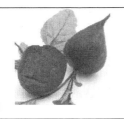

Note: Eliminate any foods on the "include" list that you suspect are problematic and do not agree with your constitution.

For more info please contact:
Anne Angelone, MS, Licensed Acupuncturist
www.anneangelone.com

The Paleo Autoimmune Protocol

Foods To Include:

Fruits:
Apples, apricots, Asian pears, bananas, blueberries, blackberry, boysenberry, cherries, cranberry, figs, grapefruit, cherries, kiwi, lemons, limes, melons, nectarine, oranges, peaches, pears, persimmons, plums, pluots, plantains, pomegranate, raspberry, strawberry.

Caution: watermelon, mango, pineapple, grapes, dried fruits, dehydrated fruits.

Fruit FODMAPs: Apples, apricots, cherries, pears, plum, persimmon, nectarines, peaches, pluots.

Vegetables:
Asparagus, arugula, artichoke, avocado, basil, beet, beet greens, broccoli, broccoli rabe, burdock, bok choy, cabbage, carrots, cauliflower, celery, chard, chicory, collards, chard, cucumber, scallion, Jerusalem

Cook broccoli cabbage cauliflower

artichoke, jicama, kale, kohlrabi, lambsquarters, leeks, lettuce, mustard, nettles, okra, onions, purslane, spinach, summer squash, turnips, artichoke hearts, Brussels sprouts, daikon radish, zucchini, fennel root, dandelion greens, red cabbage, green cabbage, Napa cabbage, water chestnuts, watercress, radish, shallot, turnips.

Vegetable FODMAPs: artichoke, asparagus, cabbage, garlic, leeks, okra, onions, snow peas, radicchio, avocado, beet root, broccoli, Brussels sprouts, mushrooms, butternut squash, pumpkin, cauliflower, celery, fennel bulb, green peas, mushrooms, sauerkraut.

Dense carbs: Beets, acorn squash, butternut squash, yams, sweet potato, taro, plantain and lotus root, cassava root, manioc, tapioca, yucca.

Dense carb FODMAPs: yams, butternut squash and sweet potatoes.

Vegetable SIBO caution: Parsnips, yams jicama, kohlrabi, okra, sweet potato, taro, plantain, Jerusalem artichoke, parsnips, and lotus root.

Fungi: Button mushrooms, portabella, oyster, chanterelle, puffball, crimini, etc.

Wild fish: Salmon, mackerel, herring, halibut, shellfish, oysters, cod, tuna, flounder, sardines, hake, skate, trout, red snapper, etc.

Meat: Beef, chicken; quail, squab, duck, goose, turkey, Cornish game hen; pasture-raised lamb, pork, buffalo/bison, goat, emu, ostrich, sausage (without fillers or nightshade spices); liver, kidney, heart, organic sliced meats (gluten, sugar free), uncured nitrate/nitrite-free deli meats and bacon from grass-fed/pastured beef/pork.

Milk and yogurt: coconut milk, unsweetened coconut yogurt.

Coconut FODMAPs: coconut milk, unsweetened coconut yogurt.

Fats: extra virgin olive oil, coconut oil, flaxseed, sesame, walnut, hazelnut oil, coconut oil, red palm oil.

Caution: nut and seed based oils: flaxseed oil, sesame oil, walnut oil, hazelnut oil, macadamia nut oil.

Coconut: coconut oil, coconut butter, coconut milk, coconut cream, unsweetened coconut yogurt, unsweetened coconut flakes, coconut aminos, coconut kefir.

Coconut FODMAPs: dried coconut, coconut flour, coconut cream, coconut milk, and coconut butter.

Beverages: filtered or distilled water, herbal tea, mineral water, broths, freshly made veggie juice, green smoothies, kombucha, kefir water, coconut kefir.

Teas: Herbal teas: Peppermint, ginger, lemongrass, spearmint, chamomile, rooibos, lavender, cinnamon, milk thistle.

Fermented foods: sauerkraut, pickles, pickled ginger, pickled cucumbers, unsweetened coconut yogurt, unsweetened coconut kefir (without corn or rice-based thickening agents), kombucha, kimchee, kefir water, pickles fermented with salt, beet kvass, lacto-fermented vegetables and fruits such as fermented beets, carrots, and green papaya.

Condiments: Apple cider vinegar, Balsamic vinegar, coconut vinegar, Red Boat fish sauce and coconut aminos.

Herbs and spices: turmeric, ginger, rosemary, basil, cilantro, garlic, ginger, lemongrass, peppermint, oregano, parsley, sage, sea, salt, thyme, tarragon, spearmint, marjoram, mace, chives, chamomile, chervil, cinnamon, bay leaves, cloves, dill, horseradish, saffron, sea salt.

Caution: black pepper, allspice, white, green and pink peppercorns, juniper, cardamom, star anise and vanilla bean.

Sugar substitutes: cinnamon, mint and ginger.

Caution: honey, maple syrup, molasses, unrefined cane sugar, and date sugar.

Superfoods to include:

Bone broth, fermented cod liver oil, gelatin, coconut yogurt, coconut oil, pastured/grass-fed organ meat e.g. liver, wild-caught cold water fish (e.g. salmon, sardines, herring, mackerel), power veggies e.g. Swiss chard, spinach, broccoli, Brussels sprouts, green smoothies (e.g. with kale, blueberries, avocado* and ginger) fermented vegetables and probiotic foods. *Note: Always consider adding a source of fat to green smoothies (like avocado, coconut oil) to aid in the absorption of fat-soluble vitamins.

Immune balancing foods to include:

Probiotics from foods like sauerkraut, coconut yogurt, kimchee, kombucha and kefir. EPA/DHA from salmon, sardines, tuna, mackerel and grass fed meats. Vitamin D from cod liver oil, herring, trout, salmon, halibut, mushrooms, beef liver and mainly sunshine! Vitamin A from liver, sweet potatoes, carrots, dark leafy greens, butternut squash, pumpkin, cod liver oil and Vitamin E from basil, oregano, olives, spinach.

Note: eliminate any food on the "include" list that does not agree with your constitution.

Foods to Eliminate:

Veggies: all nightshades.

Fruit: avoid canned fruits.

Caution: watermelon, mango, pineapple, grapes, dried fruits and dehydrated fruits

Processed and canned meats: bacon, fatty cuts of lamb, beef, pork, deli meats, smoked/dried/salted meat and fish.
Sausages and deli meats with seed-based or nightshade spices.

Fish: Whale, shark, swordfish. Farmed tilapia and catfish quantities should be moderate.

Nuts and Seeds: Avoid all nuts and seeds including almonds, Brazil nuts, cashews, chestnuts, hazelnuts, macadamias, pecans, walnuts, pine nuts, pistachios, pumpkin, and sunflower seeds and seed based spices: anise, annatto, black cumin, celery, coriander, cumin, dill, fennel, fenugreek, mustard, nutmeg, poppy, sesame.

Dairy: cow and other animal (goat/sheep) milks, cheese, cottage cheese, cream, butter, yogurt, ice-cream, non-dairy creamers, soy milk, whey, butter, cheeses, frozen desserts, mayonnaise.

Oils: margarine, butter, shortening, any processed hydrogenated oils, peanut oil, mayonnaise.

Beans and Legumes: avoid-all beans, black-eyed peas, cashews, chickpeas, lentils, miso, peas, peanuts/peanut butter, soybean and soy products.

Fungi: avoid medicinal mushrooms e.g. Shiitake, Maitake and Reishi mushrooms.

Soy: soy milk, soy sauce, tofu, tempeh, soy protein, edamame.

Drinks: sodas, fruit juice, alcoholic beverages, coffee, green, black tea, all caffeinated beverages.

Condiments: ketchup, relish, soy sauce, BBQ sauce, chutneys, other condiments, baker's and brewer's yeast.

Sweeteners: avoid white or brown sugar, high fructose corn syrup, corn syrup, fruit sweeteners, Truvia, maple syrup, agave, brown rice syrup, Splenda, Equal, Nutrasweet, Xylitol, stevia, raw green stevia.

Grains: amaranth, barley, buckwheat, corn including cornmeal and popcorn, millet, oats, oatmeal, quinoa, rice, rye, sorghum, teff, triticale, and wheat including varieties such as spelt, emmer, farro, einkorn, kamut, durum and other forms such as bulgur, cracked wheat and wheat berries.

Grain products: corn tortillas, chips, starch, syrup, noodles, cakes, breads, rolls, muffins, noodles, crackers, cookies, cake, doughnuts, pancakes, waffles, pasta, tortillas, pizza, pita, flat bread.

Grain like substances or pseudo-cereals: amaranth, buckwheat, cattail, chia, cockscomb, kañiwa, pitseed, goosefoot, quinoa, and wattleseed (aka acacia seed).

Gluten containing foods: BBQ sauce, binders, bouillon, brewer's yeast, cold cuts, condiments, emulsifiers, fillers, gum, hot dogs, hydrolyzed plant and vegetable protein, ketchup, soy sauce, lunch meats, malt, malt flavoring, malt vinegar, matzo, modified food starch, monosodium glutamate, non-dairy creamer, processed salad dressings, seitan, stabilizers, teriyaki sauce, textured vegetable protein.

Legumes: including peas, beans, lentils, soy, and peanuts.

Lectins: Avoid nuts, beans, soy, potatoes, tomato, eggplant, peppers, peanut oil, peanut butter, soy oil, etc.

Nightshade vegetables: this includes potatoes (not sweet potatoes), all tomatoes, red and green peppers, chili peppers, eggplants, tomatillos, sweet bell peppers, jalapenos, cayenne, Habanero, Anaheim and Serrano et al. peppers. Avoid chili peppers in dried powders such as paprika, chili powder, curry powder, chili pepper flakes, hot sauces, Tabasco sauces, salsas, goji berries and ashwaganda.

Dairy: all dairy products, including milk cream, cheese, from cows, goats, sheep, etc.

Eggs: or foods that contain eggs (e.g. mayonnaise).

Alcohol: all alcohol.

All processed food: cured meats, sugar, pre-mixed seasonings and sauces, mayonnaise, mustard, canned foods.

Sugars: Avoid: white or brown sugar, high fructose corn syrup, corn syrup, fruit sweeteners, Truvia, agave, brown rice syrup, Splenda, Equal, Nutrasweet, Xylitol, stevia, raw green stevia, coconut sugar and palm sugar.

Seed based spices: anise, annatto, black cumin, celery, coriander, cumin, dill, fennel, fenugreek, mustard, nutmeg, poppy, sesame, cacao.

Berry and fruit based spices: black pepper, allspice, white, green and pink peppercorns, juniper, cardamom, star anise and vanilla bean.

Coffee: Remove coffee for 30 days and proceed with caution upon reintroducing it.

Tea: Remove green and black tea for 30 days, reintroduce and note reactions.

Avoid immune stimulants: Echinacea purpurea extract, astragalus,

ashwaganda, beta glucans, chlorella,
glycyrrhiza, licorice root, goldenseal,
panax ginseng, grape seed extract,
Melissa officinalis (lemon balm),
Maitake, Reishi, Shiitake, caffeine,
green tea, coffee, lycopene, pine bark
extract, willow bark, pycnogenol,
genistein, quercetin.

Caution Foods

FODMAPS

FODMAPs: describe short-chain carbohydrates found in many common foods. FODMAPs stands for Fermentable Oligo-, Di- and Mono-saccharides, and Polyols (sugar alcohols).

FODMAPs in the autoimmune protocol: Apples, artichokes, apricots, cherries, pears, plum, persimmon, nectarines, peaches, pluots, artichoke, asparagus, cabbage, garlic, leeks, okra, onions, radicchio, avocado, beet root, broccoli, Brussels sprouts, mushrooms, butternut squash, pumpkin, cauliflower, celery, fennel bulb, mushrooms, sauerkraut, dried coconut, coconut flour, coconut milk, coconut cream, coconut butter, honey, grapes, dried fruits, blackberries, apricots.

SIBO

SIBO: Small Intestine Bacterial Overgrowth (SIBO) is now recognized as a significant yet overlooked cause of IBS.

SIBO caution foods in the autoimmune protocol: Parsnips, yams jicama, kohlrabi, okra, sweet potato, taro, plantain, Jerusalem artichoke, parsnips, lotus root, tapioca, cassava and yucca.

High Salicylate Foods

Salicylate sensitivity has the potential to create more inflammation in the body and has been linked to IBS, Crohn's and Colitis.

Salicylate Caution Foods in the autoimmune protocol: berries, apricot, avocado, blackberry, cherries, plum/prune, green olives, endive, gherkin, radish, tangelo, tangerine, water chestnut, coconut oil, olive oil, all dried fruits, honey, date, grape, guava, orange, pineapple.

High Histamine Foods

Those who have salicylate intolerance may also have histamine intolerance. Like FODMAP intolerance, Histamine intolerance may tip you off to SIBO and/or dysbiotic bacteria.

Histamine Caution Foods in the autoimmune protocol: oranges, grapefruit, lemons, lime, sauerkraut, bacon spinach, cinnamon, vinegar, shellfish, leftover meat, vinegar pickles, sauerkraut, kombucha, spinach, berries, cloves, dried fruit.

High Oxalate Foods

Foods that are high in oxalates can contribute to pain and inflammation.

High Oxalate Foods in the autoimmune protocol: sweet potatoes, endive, asparagus, Brussels sprouts, cucumbers, celery and beets, chard, beet greens.

Reintroduction of Foods:

If you have a known gluten intolerance, as most with autoimmune conditions do, proceed with caution if reintroducing these proteins as they may cause the same antibody/inflammatory reaction as gluten does: dairy proteins (casein, casomorphin, butyrophilin, and whey), oats, brewer/baker's yeast, instant coffee, sorghum, millet, corn, rice and potato.

Since reintroduction of foods may cause pronounced reactions, it's important to inform your medical practitioner about your diet and about reintroducing foods and any exacerbation of symptoms.

When reintroducing a food, do so one food at a time, wait 72 hours, note any reactions (headache, joint ache, skin rash, decreased mental clarity etc.), wait until the symptom subsides, then reintroduce the next food.

If symptoms come back after going off the protocol, you can always return to the AIP template to rapidly decrease the inflammatory response. Always check with your doctor if you have a flare up of symptoms.

About

My own experience with Ankylosing Spondylitis led me to study the underlying mechanisms of disease expression through Traditional Chinese Medicine, Nutrigenomics (how food speaks to your genes), Paleo Nutrition, and finally to Functional Medicine classes with Dr. Datis Kharrazian including Functional Blood Chemistry Analysis, Mastering the Thyroid, Neurotransmitters and the Brain, Functional Endocrinology, Autoimmunity and Gluten Sensitivity. Based on my personal and clinical experience, I believe this protocol is the perfect dietary template to halt autoimmune reactions.

For more info on the triggers and treatment of autoimmunity, please read my
e-book: The Autoimmune Paleo Plan

For more info about Autoimmune Paleo

Challenge classes contact:

Anne Angelone, Licensed
Acupuncturist
Bachelor of Science, Cornell University
Master of Science, American College of

Traditional Chinese Medicine

Member of Primal Docs
The Paleo Physician's Network
And Dr. Kharrazian's Thyroid Docs

Website: www.anneangelone.com

Dedication and Gratitude

This project is dedicated to the patients and practitioners who are spreading the word about this simple yet profound equation for halting autoimmune reactions: remove triggers; resolve intestinal permeability and silence inflammatory gene expression. The discussion about a more tailored Paleo food plan for autoimmunity was initiated by Robb Wolf in The Paleo Solution, as an autoimmune caveat to remove nightshades, eggs, nuts and seeds from the standard Paleo food plan. Diane Sanfilippo, in the phenomenal Practical Paleo, recommends and builds on this healthy template for autoimmunity, as have practitioners like Dr. Terry Wahls, Chris Kresser, L.Ac., and Dr. Datis Kharrazian who encourage similar food templates to reverse autoimmune reactions. The protocol presented here was inspired by the important work of Sarah Ballantyne, Ph.D. whose extensive knowledge and research has

contributed greatly to the current food lists and considerations in this book. For other important food and non-food aspects of the AIP, check out Sarah Ballantyne's blog, The Paleo Mom,
and book: The Paleo Approach: Reverse Autoimmune Disease and Heal Your Body.

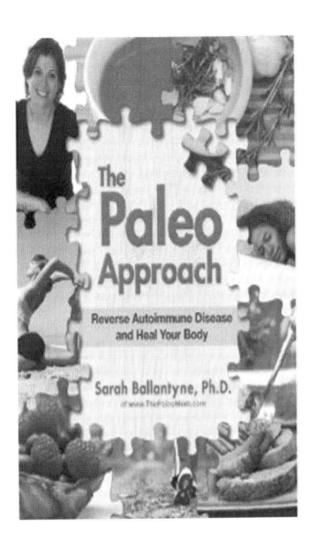

The
Paleo
Approach

Reverse Autoimmune Disease
and Heal Your Body

Sarah Ballantyne, Ph.D.
of www.ThePaleoMom.com

Autoimmune Resources:

- Sarah Ballantyne, Ph.D. aka: The Paleo Mom

- Autoimmune Paleo and You

- Autoimmune-Paleo

- Practical Paleo by Diane Sanfilippo and Balanced Bites

- Chris Kresser's: Personal Paleo Code

- The Paleo Parents Pinterest page

breakfast: Cold Salmon er Crab
½ melon

Meats/Proteins	% Protein	% Fat
Skinless turkey breast	94	5
Boiled shrimp	90	10
Orange roughy	90	10
Pollock	90	10
Broiled lobster	89	5
Red snapper	87	13
Dungeness crab	86	10
Alaskan King Crab	85	15
Buffalo roast	84	16
Broiled mackerel	82	18
Roast venison	81	19
Broiled halibut	80	20
Beef sweetbreads	77	23
Steamed clams	73	12
Pork tenderloin	72	28
Beef heart	69	30
broiled tuna	68	32
veal steak	68	32
sirloin beef steak	65	35

Made in the USA
Lexington, KY
17 May 2013